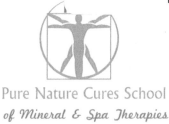

Magnesium at Home

25 Most Common Health Conditions &
How Magnesium Salts Can Help

by Galina St George

All Rights Reserved. No part of this publication may be reproduced in any form or by any means, including scanning, photocopying, or otherwise without prior written permission of the copyright holder.
Copyright © 2020

Table of Contents

Disclaimer 5
Introduction 7
Why is magnesium so important to us? 11
Causes of magnesium deficiency 14
Signs of magnesium deficiency 17
Supplementation methods 20
Magnesium products for transdermal application 25
25 Health Conditions to Address with Magnesium Salts
.... 31
   1. Stress, anxiety, irritability, sleep problems 32
2. Back Pain 36
   3. Joint pain, arthritis 41
   4. Muscle cramps, pain, tension, tremors & restless leg syndrome 44
   5. Constipation, colicky pain & stomach cramps 47
   6. Tension headaches & migraines 49
   7. Sore throat, gingivitis & mouth ulcers 51
   8. Low energy & fatigue 53
   9. Osteoporosis 55
   10. ADHD 57
   11. Fibromyalgia 60

12. High cholesterol 63
13. A link between magnesium, high blood sugar, type II diabetes, hypertension, heart disease, metabolic syndrome & obesity 67
14. Obesity, weight problems 72
15. Asthma 74
16. Magnesium for girls and women 79
17. Fertility & sexual health 84
18. Stretch marks, old scars 90
19. Heavy metal & radioactive toxicity 93
20. Sport 97
21. Allergies & chemical sensitivities 102
22. Ageing skin & wrinkles 105
23. Acne 109
24. Mental health 114
25. Cancer 117

How to Make Magnesium Oil at Home 124

Magnesium-rich foods 127

Conclusion 129

Further Information & Links 130

Disclaimer

The author of this book believes that a natural and holistic approach to health and maintaining a balance within the human body are of utmost importance in experiencing energy, vitality, and vibrant health throughout life.

This material is written for the express purpose of sharing educational information and scientific research gathered from the studies and experiences of the author, healthcare professionals, scientists, nutritionists and other informed persons.

None of the information contained in this book is intended to diagnose, prevent, treat, or cure any disease, nor is it intended to prescribe any of the techniques, materials or concepts presented as a form of treatment for any illness or medical condition.

Before beginning any work relating to health, diet or exercise, it is highly recommended that you first obtain the consent and advice of licensed health care professional.

The author assumes no responsibility for the choices you make after you review the information contained herein and your consultation with a licensed healthcare professional.

While the author of this book does everything possible to provide valid reference sources of the information cited in this book it is important to remember that unlike printed materials, online content is constantly changing. For this reason, some of the web references provided in the book may have expired due to such changes and become invalid at the time of reading. The author bears no responsibility for these changes and invalidation of the reference sources.

Introduction

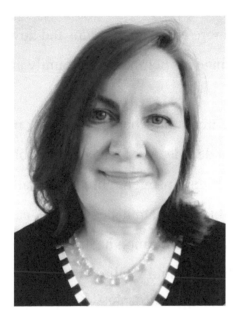

First of all, I would like to say that this book is NOT meant to be an exhaustive study of magnesium. There are other excellent books on the subject which achieve this goal – by Dr Carolyn Dean, Dr Mark Sircus, Dr Mildred Seelig, as well as some of the websites mentioned here, such as mgwater.com.

My goal was to talk about the benefits, uses and applications of magnesium salts and supplements. I also wanted to show how magnesium salts could be used to help with 25 most common health conditions. Think of it as a practical guide to help you learn more about magnesium and how you can benefit from using it to help yourself, family and friends.

I have been researching the benefits of using minerals for health for over a decade. My focus has been on learning how magnesium chloride, Epsom & Himalayan salts, as well as clays, mud, zeolite and diatomaceous earth, can help humans and animals deal with common health problems and maintain health, youth and vitality. I have also been using these wonderful nature's gifts extensively for myself and my clients.

Magnesium has always been my favourite mineral. One reason for it is its versatility regarding what it can help us with. It has certainly helped me, my family, friends and clients in many ways. Joint pain, loss of energy, frequent infections, high blood sugar level, high blood pressure, insomnia, stressed mind, leg cramps, tired aching feet, stomach cramps, constipation, wrinkles, chest pain, skin outbreaks and many other problems have been helped by using magnesium.

I have had people writing to me to say how their lives have changed as a result of using magnesium salts.

The goal of this book is to show why I am so passionate about magnesium and why it takes a special place among all the other minerals, what happens when we are deficient in it and how to correct the deficiency in a home environment. As I am writing this, I have a bottle of magnesium oil on a bookshelf – it is always with me!

In this book, I have listed 25 common problems which will benefit from magnesium supplementation. I have limited myself to this number simply because if I listed all of the conditions which require magnesium for healing, I would have to write a thick volume. While the list here is non-exhaustive, it covers the issues which have touched me or people I know at least once in a lifetime. This is the reason for the selection.

While do I cover the subject of oral and intravenous supplementation methods in this book, my focus is on how to supplement magnesium transdermally – i.e. through the skin. I have been developing treatments and writing courses on the subject of transdermal magnesium supplementation for some time since I believe that it is the safest and fastest method to top our bodies with this vital mineral.

If you want to learn more about the procedures and courses, visit https://courses.purenaturecures.com. To read more about magnesium, visit my blog – https://magnesiumoil.org.uk.

Galina St George

Pure Nature Cures
School of Mineral & Spa Therapies

Why is magnesium so important to us?

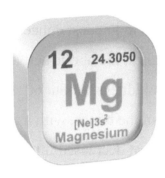

Magnesium is rightly called "the mineral of life". There are few substances which attract so much attention and instigate so much scientific research. The reason is that not only magnesium participates in over 300 biochemical reactions in the body, but it also helps to maintain normal muscle and nerve function, steady heart rhythm, optimal blood pressure, healthy immune system, strong bones and normal blood sugar level. It plays a vital role in preventing heart disease, diabetes, cancer, osteoporosis and a whole range of other dangerous and debilitating conditions.

Following potassium, magnesium is the second most abundant intracellular cation in the human body and the fourth most abundant mineral in the body overall. The average 70kg human body contains about 24g of magnesium. It is found in greatest concentrations in the tissues having the highest metabolic activity, such as the heart, liver, brain and kidneys. About 60% of the total body magnesium is found in the bones, with a third of it acting as a reserve for the times of decreased intake and increased utilisation. Its function is to maintain stable serum magnesium levels. The remainder of magnesium is found mostly inside the cells of other tissues. Only 1% is found in the blood where it plays a vital role, so the body works very hard to keep the blood magnesium level constant.

"[Magnesium is an]...important participant in enzyme processes which ensure protein biosynthesis and carbohydrate metabolism. It is also very important for the nervous and muscular systems, helps to maintain the healthy tone of the blood vessels. Magnesium is a 'calming' element for the nervous system slowing down the brain activity. It expands the blood vessels and is a natural diuretic. Generally, it is vital for all body systems and processes.

The adult requirement in magnesium is 350-500mg per day. Fresh green vegetables, seafood, soybeans, special nutritional yeasts, seeds, apples and whole grains are rich sources."

http://www.traceminerals.com/research/magnesium.html

Causes of magnesium deficiency

The following are some of the factors which cause magnesium deficiency:

- Stress – physical and mental

- Certain medications (e.g. insulin, diuretics, some asthma medications, birth control pills, corticosteroids, blood pressure control medicines)

- Extreme physical training

- Chemical toxins getting into the body from the environment (e.g. fertilisers, herbicides)

- Excessive intake of sodium chloride (table salt), sugar, caffeine, alcohol, nicotine, cocaine, fizzy drinks (especially colas)

- Prolonged intense sweating, due to exercise or illness
- Diarrhoea
- Consumption of junk food and drinks
- Consuming food products which come from magnesium-deficient soils
- Drinking water which is high in potassium
- Prolonged physical exercise
- Diabetes
- Obesity
- Kidney disease
- Malabsorption – this can be due to compromised levels of enzymes, or unhealthy condition of the gut
- Digestive disorders
- Crohn's disease

- Chemotherapy and radiotherapy
- Liver disease
- Inflammation
- Serious injuries
- Excessive intake of vitamin D
- Excessive consumption of dairy products (especially cheese)
- Pancreatitis
- Severe burns.

Signs of magnesium deficiency

Magnesium deficiency is hard to diagnose through blood tests since very little of it is found in the blood. However, low overall magnesium level shows itself in various symptoms that we need to look out for. Early signs of magnesium deficiency include:

- Loss of appetite
- Feeling stressed & anxious
- Feeling constantly tired & weak
- Painful joints
- Tense, painful muscles
- Spots and acne
- High blood sugar
- Inability to lose weight

- Nausea

- Headaches

- Weight gain

- Muscle cramps

- Heart palpitations

- Spasms in the chest

- Leg cramps

- Constipation and stomach cramps

- Inability to have a good night's sleep.

Dr Carolyn Dean lists the following conditions which develop in cases of magnesium deficiency or and require magnesium supplementation:

"Acid reflux, Adrenal fatigue, Alzheimer's disease, Angina, Anxiety and panic attacks, Arthritis, Asthma, Atherosclerosis, Blood clots, Bowel disease, Brain dysfunction, Bruxism or teeth grinding, Cholesterol elevation, cystitis, Depression, Detoxification, Diabetes, Fatigue, Headaches, Heart disease, Hypertension, Hypoglycemia, Indigestion, Inflammation, Insomnia, IBS, Kidney disease, Kidney stones, Migraine, Musculo-skeletal conditions: (muscle cramps, fibrositis, fibromyalgia, GI spasms, tension headaches, muscle spasms or muscle contractions in any muscle of the body, chronic neck and back pain, jaw tension), Nerve problems – Neuralgia, Neuritis, Neuropathy (burning pain, muscle weakness, numbness paralysis, pins and needles, seizures and convulsions, tingling twitching, vertigo, confusion), Obstetrical and gynecological problems (PMS, dysmenorrhea, female infertility, premature contractions, preeclampsia and eclampsia, cerebral palsy, sudden infant death syndrome, male infertility), Osteoporosis, Parkinson's disease, Raynaud's syndrome, Sports injuries, Sports recovery, Tempromandibular joint syndrome, Tongue biting, Tooth decay." http://drcarolyndean.com

To find out if it is magnesium deficiency that is causing any of the above symptoms, take oral magnesium supplements or use transdermal top-up methods and watch for how your body responds to it. If you start experiencing improvements, it could mean that you were deficient.

Supplementation methods

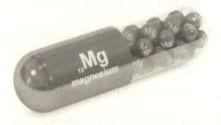

There are 3 methods of magnesium supplementation – oral (by mouth), intravenous (through the skin) and transdermal (through the skin).

Oral supplementation is used by most people. While some such supplements are effective, others are not as much. For example, magnesium oxide requires stomach acid to be absorbed. This can upset digestion, especially in cases where the digestive system is already compromised, as in cases where stomach acidity is low. So the stomach acid needed for digestion is used to break down magnesium oxide, which may leave a person with symptoms of indigestion, such as gas, bloating, heaviness in the stomach and even diarrhoea. So while magnesium oxide is relatively cheap, it is not the best one to take. Invest in chelated magnesium supplements such as magnesium citrate, magnesium glycinate, magnesium orotate, magnesium threonate, magnesium taurate, magnesium maleate and chelated magnesium including amino acids and proteins.

Magnesium chloride and magnesium sulphate are salt-based forms of magnesium which are easily absorbed when hydrated since salts split into ions in water. They can be taken internally too – with caution. People with kidney problems should speak to their GP before introducing magnesium salts to their diet. The same applies to people who are taking any kind of medication.

Generally, oral is the least effective method of magnesium supplementation of the three listed options. The reason is that magnesium from oral supplements gets absorbed in the small intestine, and people with the compromised digestive system and clogged up intestinal tract absorption of magnesium becomes ineffective. Moreover, even chelated magnesium may cause diarrhoea in some people. This means that much of magnesium from supplements does not get absorbed and benefit the body. Only 35-40% of magnesium gets absorbed by the body from oral supplements. This does not mean that oral supplementation should not be an option. It simply means that it needs to be used in conjunction with other forms of supplementation, such as transdermal.

Injecting magnesium intravenously is the fastest and most effective supplementation method. It is used to in hospitals to help stop a cardiac arrest for example. It is also used for patients undergoing angioplasty, or those suffering from arrhythmia, asthma and diabetes. Both magnesium chloride and magnesium sulphate solutions are being used in these procedures.

"Magnesium's powerful vasodilator action immediately became apparent with its action increasing in potency with

increased initial blood concentrations. After magnesium infusions, there is a significant increase in cardiac output, and the cardiac index is maintained at a higher level than that of control groups during the induction of anaesthesia and endotracheal intubation."
http://drsircus.com/general/magnesium-administration/#_edn5

However, intravenous magnesium injections, despite all their power, life-saving advantages, have a major disadvantage – they can only be administered in a clinic, under medical observation, and not in a home environment by an unqualified person.

Transdermal supplementation is fast becoming the most convenient option for many people, due to its simplicity, versatile applications and fast results. Transdermal magnesium supplementation is based on the ability of the skin to absorb. In cases of transdermal applications, the skin absorbs ions of magnesium from saline solutions of magnesium chloride and magnesium sulphate.

Unlike oral and intravenous forms of supplementation, transdermal applications of magnesium salts are relatively safe. The reason for it is that the skin acts as a barrier to excessive amounts of magnesium ions, which means that this form of supplementation is fast but gradual and gentle giving the body the amount that it needs, which not only reduces the risk of overdosing but also the load on excretory organs such as the kidneys. Apart from that, transdermal applications of magnesium salts bring about physical and mental relaxation and pain relief within minutes, which is undoubtedly beneficial to most people living a fast-paced life or suffering from painful conditions.

To some people applying magnesium solutions on the skin – for example in the form of magnesium oil – can be a bit uncomfortable at first. However, this can be managed by diluting the solution further if necessary. This minor itch is undoubtedly outweighed by multiple benefits of such applications. You just get used to it eventually.

Magnesium products for transdermal application

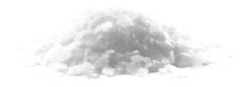

Transdermal applications involve the following products:

- **Magnesium chloride salt flakes** – also called magnesium chloride hexahydrate due to it containing 6 molecules of water. The flakes are highly hygroscopic (they absorb water easily), so need to be kept in a dry place. A high temperature will melt the flakes into a watery mass due to the water content, so it is important to keep them in a relatively cool environment.

- **Magnesium oil** – this is not actually an oil, but a highly concentrated magnesium chloride solution which has a consistency and feel of an oil. This makes it easy to apply on the skin by hand. Some people prefer to spray it on, which is also fine.

- **Magnesium gel** – this includes magnesium chloride and a gel component which makes the product gentler on the skin, so people with sensitive skin may prefer it to magnesium oil.

- **Magnesium sulphate, or Epsom salt** – otherwise called magnesium sulphate heptahydrate. The salt contains 7 molecules of water, so is also vulnerable to warm temperatures. It is also highly hygroscopic and needs to be kept in a dry place, just like magnesium chloride.

- **Dead Sea salt** is very rich in magnesium. Much of magnesium chloride comes from the Dead Sea. This salt has long been used with fantastic results. Due to its high content of magnesium chloride, it should also be kept in a dry cool place.

Methods of transdermal magnesium supplementation include:

- **Magnesium oil rub (spray)** includes rubbing the body or parts of it with magnesium oil. Since it is so easily spread, you will only need a small amount of it for a rub. Spraying it on is another application method which some find more convenient, especially with the areas which are difficult to reach by hand, such as the back. If possible, I would still suggest asking someone to rub it around even after it has been sprayed, to ensure even distribution.

- **Magnesium oil massage** is normally done by another person. The whole body is being massaged with magnesium oil. This is a luxurious, very relaxing treatment with an added benefit of a massage, so if at all possible, ask a family member to do it for you or book a treatment with a therapist.

- **Bath** – add 300-500g of magnesium chloride, Epsom salt or Dead Sea salt crystals to a bath of warm water. Take daily if possible, or at least once a week. In times of stress, or if you have a chronic condition which involves anxiety, pain, fatigue, chronic headaches and similar problems, take as required. Adding more salt will strengthen the effect.

- **Footbath** is a cheaper and faster alternative to a full-body bath. Although it is not as effective in terms of the effect on the whole body as a bath, it is still a powerful treatment which helps to deliver magnesium to the body quickly through the feet. It is very relaxing and works wonders for tired feet, as well as a stressed mind. It's good to take a foot bath just before going to bed due to its sleep-inducing effect. You would need 150-200g of magnesium chloride, Epsom salt of Dead Sea salt per a foot bath (about 5 litres of warm water). Take as needed, even every day.

- **Compress** – could be an answer to local problems, such as joint pain, muscle tension, contusions, bruises, ulcers, etc. You will need to mix magnesium salt in warm water at about 1:5 ratio. Soak a cloth, squeeze it slightly, apply on the area, wrap with cling film, then with a plastic sheet or compress paper, and finally a warm scarf around the area. Leave on for up to 2 hours, or even overnight.

- **Body wrap** – this can be done with or without heat, depending on the temperature. I have developed a Far Infrared Thermal Magnesium Wrap which you may read about on the website of the school which I run –

https://courses.purenaturecures.com. Anybody can learn how to do the treatment once they sign up to the course. The treatment can be used for a variety of conditions, and all the 25 conditions listed below.

- **Mouth wash** – add 1 tablespoonful of magnesium chloride to about 250ml of warm water. Rinse as required. The advantage of this rinse compared to a sodium chloride solution is that magnesium chloride does not damage tissues which it is in contact with, while sodium chloride does.

25 Health Conditions to Address with Magnesium Salts

1. Stress, anxiety, irritability, sleep problems

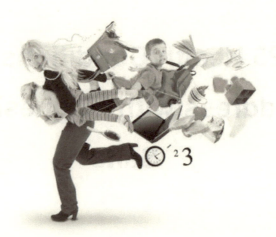

Stress depletes magnesium levels because the stress response uses up a lot of body energy and resources. When we are under stress we are often anxious and irritable which is often accompanied by sleep problems.

Magnesium is one of the most powerful natural relaxants acting in a calming way on the nervous system. In challenging times it is very important to increase magnesium supplementation, both by taking magnesium supplements and by using various magnesium-based procedures. I would suggest adding a good strength vitamin B complex to it, as well as zinc, selenium, calcium and vitamin D.

Apart from using up most of the magnesium reserves, with chronic stress, the body starts producing too much cortisol (a hormone which helps the body adjust to stress), side-effects of which include chronic inflammation, raised blood sugar level and production and release of extra insulin, which increases the risk of diabetes.

A study researching a link between stress, magnesium deficiency and immune response has found out that "Mg deficiency results in a stress effect and increased susceptibility to physiological damage produced by stress. Stress activates the sympathetic nervous system and renin-angiotensin-aldosterone axis resulting in increased oxidative stress. Aldosteronism is immunostimulatory, as is commonly seen in congestive heart failure. The inflammatory syndrome induces mechanisms dependent on cytosolic calcium activation. These interrelationships support that the Mg effect on intracellular calcium homeostasis may be a

common link between stress and inflammation".
http://www.omicsonline.org/magnesium-influence-on-stress-and-immune-function-in-exercise-2161-0673.1000111.pdf

High cholesterol level and formation of arterial deposits on the walls are almost inevitable in cases of prolonged stress. Comfort eating contributes to weight gain, which in turn increases the risk of diabetes, heart disease and cancer. So it becomes a vicious circle which with time gets harder and harder to break.

It is amazing how simply by including magnesium in the diet things begin to turn for the better. Of course, magnesium alone won't do it. We need to take a whole range of steps to break this cycle and regain our health. Exercise, good nutrition, plenty of water, learning to deal with stressful situations and creating a stress-free environment at home and at work all need to be considered. But topping up magnesium levels in the body will bring almost immediate relief (depending on the method of supplementation).

Doctors have known and used magnesium (and still do) to pull a person from an emergency, such as an irregular heartbeat or heart attack, by injecting magnesium intravenously. This is a lifesaver for dying patients. So why not use this relatively cheap and very effective mineral to help ourselves which would help us avoid emergencies?

The fastest way to reduce symptoms of stress is to apply magnesium on the skin by hand, as a spray, take a magnesium bath or a foot bath. It is important to do it regularly, at least twice a week under normal conditions, and daily when under stress. I suggest taking a warm magnesium bath or a foot bath about half an hour before bedtime, since both induce profound relaxation and would make you want to sleep, which is great for those who have problems sleeping.

2. Back Pain

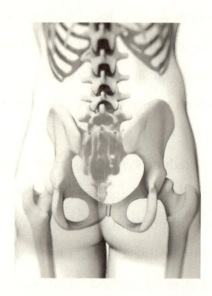

It is estimated that 80% of people in the Western world will experience lower back pain at some point in their lives. The indirect cost to the economy is estimated in hundreds of billions. The cost in human suffering is impossible to calculate.

There are 5 main reasons for commonly occurring back pain:

1. Weight issues
2. Stress
3. Long-standing psychological problems
4. Sedentary lifestyle
5. Magnesium deficiency.

Traditional medical treatment of lower back pain involves prescribing non-steroidal anti-inflammatory drugs (NSAIDs) and even opioids. Both of these, while bringing immediate pain relief, have serious side-effects while addressing only symptoms of the problem and not the cause of it. For example, NSAIDs can result in 2 to 4-times higher rate of heart attacks and strokes, digestive problems, high blood pressure, kidney problems and other issues.

Opioids, on the other hand, are highly addictive. Anti-inflammatory drugs such as aspirin, ibuprofen affect the stomach lining and often lead to digestive problems which may even result in internal bleeding. There are other medicines, often very expensive, which have even more serious consequences.

How can you help yourself?

1. **Lose weight**. Shedding even a few pounds will take a considerable load off your spine and muscles supporting it. It will also help preserve the intervertebral discs which get squashed when under extra pressure. Work towards establishing and maintaining an optimal weight to height ratio (BMI).

2. **Reduce the amount of acute and chronic stress in your life**. Identify and work towards eliminating causes of stress. You may need to ask for help from a stress management coach.

3. **Address emotional issues**. It is believed that emotional pain translates into physical problems, and back/muscle/joint pain takes the worst of it. Often when emotional issues get resolved, the pain eventually goes away.

4. **Move around more, adjust your posture**. Sedentary lifestyle, incorrect posture and repetitive strain can

result in permanent damage to the spine. Make sure that your back is supported. Sit straight, with the stomach sucked in. Take regular breaks during work.

5. **Exercise.** Gentle stretching – for example, Yoga and Pilates - is perhaps the best form of keeping the back in a good condition.

6. **Have regular massage treatments**. It will soften the tissues and help stretch the muscles.

7. **Drink lots of water**. It helps to keep muscles and joints supple and maintain intervertebral discs in a healthy state.

8. **Address magnesium deficiency** by supplementing magnesium in your diet. If magnesium is deficient, soft tissues begin to calcify and calcium crystals begin to form in joints, which contributes further to back pain. Transdermal magnesium therapy will help to soften those hardened, tense muscles and rigid joints. Take a bath with magnesium salts, apply magnesium oil on the body every day, have hot compresses. If you would like to experience fast relief

from back pain, have a Far Infrared Magnesium Wrap.

I don't want to oversimplify the issue of back pain. Some cases are complex and require a complex approach. Sometimes, when the damage has already been done, pain relief medication is unavoidable. However, even in such cases, magnesium salts can be of tremendous benefit in alleviating the worst of the pain, thus reducing our reliance on medicines.

3. Joint pain, arthritis

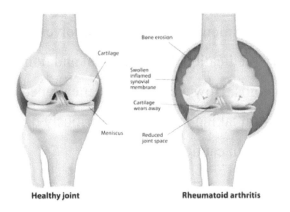

RHEUMATOID ARTHRITIS

Healthy joint — Rheumatoid arthritis

Most people experience joint pain at least once in their lifetime. It is sometimes caused by an accident, a turn in a wrong direction, and in less fortunate cases – dislocation of a joint, or a fall. For most people, joint pain heals by itself relatively quickly.

When the same joint gets injured repeatedly, the pain can become chronic. Often chronic pain is associated with chronic arthritis which can become inflammatory. This results in more pain, a swollen hot joint and loss of mobility for an affected joint. Arthritis is most commonly found in knee and hip joints, but can also be present in other joints – for example in wrists and fingers.

Medical care of patients with arthritis involves anti-inflammatory medication, both steroidal and non-steroidal, as well as opioids. However, as I have mentioned earlier, side effects from taking them can be seriously damaging to health, so use with caution.

Magnesium promotes relaxation of all tissues, including muscles and nerves. Being an anti-oxidant, it also has an anti-inflammatory action helping to protect the cartilage from further damage.

The other reason to use magnesium is to prevent deposition of calcium in the joints. Calcium by itself is damaging to the bones and joints and need magnesium to be of use to us. Moreover, oral magnesium supplementation will reduce the damaging effects of anti-inflammatory medication such as ibuprofen and aspirin.

How can you help yourself?

Transdermal magnesium applications work best in cases of joint pain and arthritis. If a joint is inflamed, rub magnesium oil over it. A cool compress could be another option, as well as a magnesium bath. Where there is no inflammation present, a very warm compress, a bath or a Far Infrared wrap could bring fast relief.

4. Muscle cramps, pain, tension, tremors & restless leg syndrome

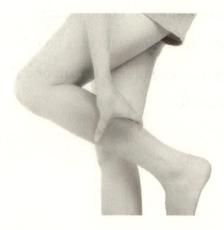

Magnesium is a crucial mineral which ensures nerve transmission. It also regulates calcium levels in tissues and blood. Calcium ensures muscle contraction, while magnesium is responsible for their release. If you suffer from muscle problems such as pain, tension, cramps, convulsions, tremors and restless leg syndrome, you are very possibly deficient in magnesium and have too much calcium circulating in the body. Insufficient magnesium also causes a build-up of lactic acid in tissues, which results in sore muscles. While magnesium supplementation often relieves the problem, it is still important to get a proper medical diagnosis to exclude any serious conditions.

While in the past it was said that the calcium to magnesium ratio should be 2:1, research has shown that a 1:1 ratio is correct. So if you take magnesium as a supplement, make sure that you take equal amounts of elemental calcium and magnesium.

How can you help yourself?

Using magnesium salts transdermally is the fastest and most effective way to reach a balance between calcium and magnesium levels. Apply magnesium oil to sore muscles and joints regularly – either by hand or as a spray. Take a bath daily – as part of the routine, or as the main procedure. A foot bath is good too, but less effective than magnesium oil applications or a full-body bath. Magnesium massage performed daily is an excellent way to relieve aches, pain and deliver necessary amounts of magnesium to the body. And finally, perhaps the most effective and fastest way to address the problem is by using a Far Infrared Magnesium

Wrap. This can be done to the whole body or affected parts.

5. Constipation, colicky pain & stomach cramps

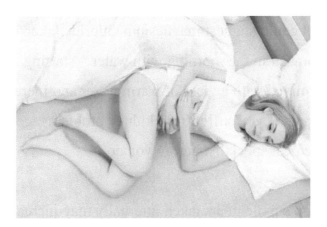

First of all, any symptoms of this kind must be investigated and diagnosed to ensure that they are not connected with serious problems which require urgent medical treatment.

If however these issues are caused by an emotional upset, insufficient activity, low water intake or incorrect nutrition, you may need to look into making appropriate changes where they are needed, with or without specialist help.

How can you help yourself?

If you suffer from constipation, remember to drink plenty of water, exercise and increase intake of fibre-rich food. Magnesium supplements taken regularly can help to loosen the stool. I could suggest magnesium chloride taken on an empty stomach in the morning with water – starting from 1 teaspoon mixed with a glass of warm water and increasing to 1 tablespoon. If you suffer from kidney problems, get advice from a medical specialist before you do it.

Magnesium supplements taken internally may increase colicky pain and cramps due to their activity in the digestive tract, so I would suggest applying magnesium oil on the stomach instead. Adding a few drops of peppermint essential oil to the mix could help even more.

Taking a magnesium bath will deliver magnesium to the body quickly and relax the digestive tract, thus hopefully reducing pain and discomfort. Every case is different though, and you may need to try various methods before you find what suits you best.

6. Tension headaches & migraines

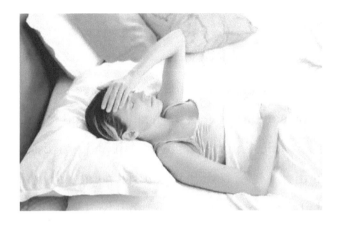

Headaches and migraines are often a result of magnesium deficiency which could lead to muscle spasms in the neck and the head. Of course, there can be a variety of reasons, so it is important to get diagnosed as soon as possible. Nevertheless, magnesium supplementation could bring relief in cases of headaches and migraine, whatever the cause.

How can you help yourself?

The fastest way to relieve these symptoms would be to apply magnesium oil on the forehead, the temples, back of the head, neck, shoulders and the scalp, and then rest in a dark cool room as long as necessary. Remember to drink plenty of water, since dehydration should be avoided to keep the symptoms away.

You may also decide to do a food intolerance test since certain foods can be triggers for headaches and migraines with some people. Cut down sugar, salt and processed food from your diet. Make sure that you sleep enough hours and go to bed at the same time – preferably by 11 pm - to get the sleep hormone melatonin in sufficient doses. Identify sources of stress and deal with them. Take a good vitamin B supplement. Gingko Biloba has been researched to improve circulation in the brain, so could be worth considering.

Have a regular magnesium massage, spray or rub magnesium oil on the body or take magnesium baths regularly to prevent headaches from coming back in the future.

7. Sore throat, gingivitis & mouth ulcers

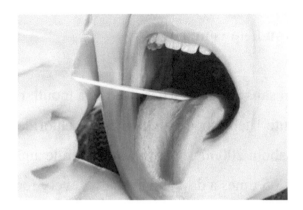

A sore throat is most commonly associated with a cold and flu infection but is sometimes a symptom of a more serious problem, so if it persists, get it checked out.

Gingivitis is a painful condition which involves inflammation of the gums which is often accompanied by bleeding. It is one of the most common causes and consequences of dental health problems. If untreated, it may lead to loss of teeth and chronic gum problems.

Mouth ulcers can have many causes and should always be medically diagnosed.

How can you help yourself?

Magnesium salts are great when used as a mouth rinse and a gargle. Dilute 1 tablespoon of magnesium chloride or Dead Sea salt in about 200ml of warm water. Gargle and rinse the mouth about 5 times a day, and also after every food intake. Unlike sodium chloride salt, magnesium salts don't damage tissues, acting in a gentle but healing way. Adding 3 drops of tea tree oil to the mix will enhance the effect of the solution. Identify what causes mouth ulcers and deal with them using a complex of measures. Get them diagnosed first though.

8. Low energy & fatigue

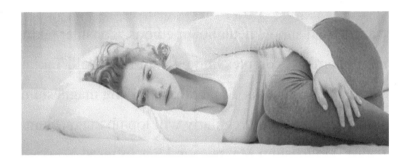

Magnesium takes a major part in energy production acting as a spark in the powerhouse of the cell – the ATP molecule. When we are deficient in magnesium, energy production slows down. This is a short explanation of why we feel tired when we suffer from magnesium deficiency.

Low energy is not only debilitating but can also be linked to other problems such as depression, weight gain, muscle and joint pain and general deterioration of health. Sometimes low energy is a result of a chronic condition, such as fibromyalgia or chronic fatigue syndrome. Get it investigated with your medical doctor.

How can you help yourself?

To boost magnesium in the body, I suggest using both oral and transdermal supplementation methods. Consider taking calcium, vitamin B complex and vitamin D as well. Taking regular magnesium baths, foot baths, applying magnesium oil by hand or as a spray regularly will top up magnesium levels fast. Magnesium Massage and Far Infrared magnesium wrap are other very effective methods to ensure quick supplementation of this energy-boosting mineral.

9. Osteoporosis

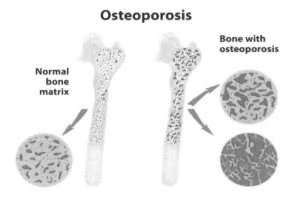

As has been mentioned already at the beginning, 60% of magnesium is found in bones. 35% of it is the reserve used by the body to support magnesium-dependent processes in the body. As we age, magnesium in the body and bones gets depleted which leads to a calcium-magnesium imbalance.

"A tight control of magnesium homeostasis seems to be crucial for bone health. Based on experimental and epidemiological studies, both low and high magnesium have harmful effects on the bones. Magnesium deficiency contributes to osteoporosis directly by acting on crystal

formation and bone cells and indirectly by impacting on the secretion and the activity of parathyroid hormone and by promoting low-grade inflammation. Less is known about the mechanisms responsible for the mineralization defects observed when magnesium is elevated. Overall, controlling and maintaining magnesium homeostasis represents a helpful intervention to maintain bone integrity."
https://www.ncbi.nlm.nih.gov/pmc/articles/PMC3775240/

How can you help yourself?

While sufficient magnesium is vital for maintaining bone health, it is also necessary to ensure that vitamins A, B, C, E and minerals such as copper, zinc, selenium, phytoestrogens and flavonoids are consumed in sufficient amounts, preferably in a food form. Regular exercise is also very important for maintaining bone density. To ensure adequate levels of magnesium in bones, apply magnesium oil daily by hand or as a spray and take magnesium baths as often as possible.

10. ADHD

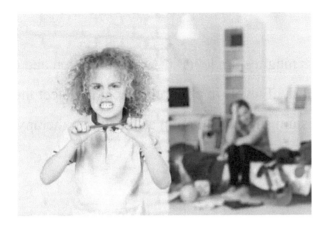

ADHD is an abbreviation for Attention Deficit Hyperactivity Disorder – a neuropsychiatric condition which is characterised by mineral deficiency. The symptoms include deficits of attention, focus, emotional instability, hyperactivity which all lead to impairment of social and professional life. ADHD is normally an early onset condition, which is why when we talk about it we almost always mention children.

Various scientific studies have discovered that most ADHD patients suffer from magnesium deficiency. Here are results of one of such studies.

"To assess magnesium level in ADHD children and compare it to the normal levels in children. Then, to detect the effect of magnesium supplementation as an add on therapy, on magnesium-deficient patients.

Methods

The study was conducted on 25 patients with ADHD and 25 controls. All subjects had magnesium estimation in serum and hair. ADHD children were further assessed by Wechsler intelligence scale for children, Conners' parent rating scale, and Wisconsin card sorting test. Then magnesium-deficient patients were assigned into 2 groups, those who received magnesium, and those who did not. The difference between the studied groups was assessed by Conners' parents' rating scale and Wisconsin card sorting test results.

Magnesium deficiency was found in 18 (72%) of ADHD

children. The magnesium supplemented group improved as regards cognitive functions as measured by the Wisconsin card sorting test and Conners' rating scale. The patients reported minor side effects from magnesium supplementation.

Conclusion

Magnesium supplementation in ADHD proves its value and safety."

http://www.sciencedirect.com/science/article/pii/S1110863015000555

How can you help your child?

There is a lot of anecdotal evidence that Epsom Salt baths act in a calming way on ADHD children and gradually improve their general condition and ability to concentrate. To make an Epsom salt bath, use 500g of salt in a bath of warm water. Such a bath can be taken daily, before bedtime. It is also important to ensure sufficient intake of the vitamin

B complex, as well as omega-3 and omega-6 oils.

11. Fibromyalgia

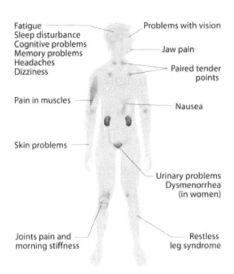

Also known as FMS, fibromyalgia is a chronic condition of an unknown origin which is characterised by muscle and joint pain and stiffness, fatigue, headaches, difficulty sleeping, IBS (Irritable Bowel Syndrome) and problems with mental concentration and memory. It is a debilitating condition which makes it impossible for sufferers to live a normal, active life.

Triggers for FMS could include stressful events, such as an illness or death of a relative, childbirth, having an operation, relationship breakdown and even an injection.

Research has established a connection between fibromyalgia and magnesium deficiency. Some suggest a possibility of misdiagnosis since severe magnesium deficiency causes symptoms similar to those of fibromyalgia.

Results of one study concluded that "transdermal MgCl2 applied twice daily on upper and lower limbs may be beneficial for patients with fibromyalgia. To our knowledge, this is the first study evaluating the effectiveness and feasibility of transdermal MgCl2 for treatment of fibromyalgia symptoms."
http://www.jcimjournal.com/jim/FullText2.aspx?articleID=S2095-4964(15)60195-9

How can you help yourself?

Apart from oral, transdermal magnesium supplementation by rubbing magnesium oil on the skin, having a magnesium massage or Far Infrared magnesium wrap will help to deliver adequate amounts of magnesium to the body fast and will help to relieve pain, increase energy levels and concentration. Regular magnesium baths are also very beneficial.

12. High cholesterol

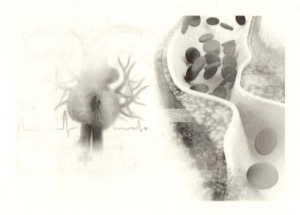

Cholesterol is a substance consisting of fat and protein which is mostly made by the liver. There are two types of cholesterol – LDL (low-density lipoprotein) and HDL (high-density lipoprotein). It is the first one which takes part in cholesterol plaque formation. HDL plays an important role by taking LDL from parts of the body where there is too much of it back to the liver. So we need HDL to keep our arteries clean and free from deadly plaque.

Cholesterol is measured via a blood test. High blood LDL is both a cause and a symptom of various problems, such as atherosclerosis, heart disease, high blood pressure and diabetes. It is therefore in our interests to keep LDL level low and HDL level high.

Clinical treatment of high cholesterol includes prescribing statins. While lowering the LDL level, statins have many adverse side-effects which can lead to more health problems and as a result to worsening of the symptoms being treated.

I have come across the following article which shows how magnesium inhibits bad cholesterol-raising the good one while having no side-effects of statins. I suggest you read it from beginning to end, especially if you are concerned about your bad cholesterol level.

"Since $Mg(2+)$-ATP is the controlling factor for the rate-limiting enzyme in the cholesterol biosynthesis sequence that is targeted by the statin pharmaceutical drugs, comparison of the effects of $Mg(2+)$ on lipoproteins with those of the statin drugs is warranted. Formation of cholesterol in the blood, as well as of cholesterol required in hormone synthesis, and membrane maintenance, is achieved in a series of enzymatic reactions that convert HMG-CoA to cholesterol. The rate-limiting reaction of this pathway is the enzymatic conversion of HMG CoA to mevalonate via HMG CoA. The statins and Mg inhibit that enzyme. Large trials have consistently shown that statins, taken by subjects with high LDL-cholesterol (LDL-C) values, lower its blood levels 35 to 65%. They also reduce the incidence of heart attacks, angina and other nonfatal cardiac events, as well as cardiac, stroke, and total mortality. These effects of statins derive less from their lowering of LDL-C than from their reduction of mevalonate formation which improves endothelial function, inhibits proliferation and migration of vascular smooth muscle cells and macrophages, promotes plaque stabilization and regression, and reduces inflammation, **Mg has effects that parallel those of statins.** For example, the enzyme that deactivates HMG-CoA Reductase requires Mg, making Mg a Reductase controller rather than an inhibitor. Mg is also necessary for the activity of lecithin cholesterol acyltransferase (LCAT), which lowers LDL-C and triglyceride levels and raises HDL-C levels. Desaturase is another Mg-dependent enzyme involved in lipid metabolism which statins do not directly affect. Desaturase catalyzes the first step in the conversion of essential fatty acids (omega-3 linoleic acid and omega-6 linolenic acid) into prostaglandins, important in cardiovascular and overall health. Mg at optimal cellular concentration is well accepted as a natural calcium channel blocker. More recent work shows that Mg also acts as a statin."

https://www.ncbi.nlm.nih.gov/pubmed/15466951

How can you help yourself?

To help reduce LDL and raise HDL levels in the blood, both oral and transdermal supplementation methods need to be considered. For transdermal supplementation, apply magnesium oil by hand, as a spray, have a regular magnesium oil massage or Far Infrared Magnesium wrap treatments. Magnesium baths and foot baths will also be beneficial.

13. A link between magnesium, high blood sugar, type II diabetes, hypertension, heart disease, metabolic syndrome & obesity

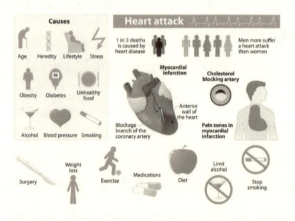

Magnesium plays a major role in regulating blood sugar level. It does so by controlling glucose and sugar metabolism. It also activates tyrosine kinase – an enzyme which is required to ensure optimal functioning of insulin receptors. In turn, insulin ensures delivery of magnesium from extracellular to intracellular compartments where it is needed for energy production. So as we can see, the magnesium-insulin interaction goes both ways, and both of them need each other to ensure our survival.

Kidneys deplete magnesium by excreting it from the body. Many people who have insulin resistance also have too much magnesium being excreted through the kidneys. A reduction of magnesium in the cells (intracellular magnesium) makes insulin resistance worse. So it becomes a vicious circle. Moreover, magnesium depletion has been linked to the progression of retinopathy in Type I and II diabetes.

Reduction of intracellular magnesium in the body and strengthening of insulin resistance leads to a depletion of the cells' ability to produce energy, which results in many health problems, including the Metabolic Syndrome and ultimately a higher risk of obesity. Moreover, insulin regulates cholesterol levels, so when magnesium is deficient, the LDL cholesterol level in the blood goes up, which if left unchecked can lead to atherosclerosis, hypertension and heart disease. It is impossible not to see how everything is connected in our body.

Here is an abstract from an article which demonstrates interconnection between magnesium, regulation of blood sugar level and type II diabetes:

"Type 2 diabetes is frequently associated with both extracellular and intracellular magnesium (Mg) deficits. A chronic latent Mg deficit or overt clinical hypomagnesemia is common in patients with type 2 diabetes, especially in those with poorly controlled glycemic profiles. Insulin and glucose are important regulators of Mg metabolism. Intracellular Mg plays a key role in regulating insulin action, insulin-mediated-glucose-uptake and vascular tone. Reduced intracellular Mg concentrations result in a defective tyrosine-kinase activity, postreceptorial impairment in insulin action and worsening of insulin resistance in diabetic patients. A low Mg intake and an increased Mg urinary loss appear the most important mechanisms that may favor Mg depletion in patients with type 2 diabetes. Low dietary Mg intake has been related to the development of type 2 diabetes and metabolic syndrome."
https://www.ncbi.nlm.nih.gov/pmc/articles/PMC4549665/

Supplementation with magnesium, especially transdermally, leads to inspiring results. "Increased magnesium intake is associated with decreased risk of developing type 2 diabetes in populations. In a prospective study of almost 85,000 women, the relative risk of diabetes for women in the highest quintile of magnesium consumption was 0.68 when compared with women in the lowest quintile.

Higher dietary intake of magnesium was among the factors associated with a reduced risk of stroke in men with hypertension. In a survey of almost 45,000 men ages 40 to 75, the overall risk of stroke was significantly lower for men in the highest quintile of intake of potassium, magnesium, and cereal fiber, but not of calcium, compared with men in the lowest quintile of intake.

A similar relationship was reported this year by Meyer and colleagues, who observed that a diet rich in magnesium, grains, fruits, and vegetables reduced the likelihood of developing type 2 diabetes in a group of almost 36,000 women.

While no consistent effect of magnesium on blood pressure has been noted among persons with diabetes, a significant blood pressure reduction was noted in diabetic patients with hypertension after dietary sodium was replaced with potassium and magnesium. In a study from Taiwan, the risk of dying from diabetes was inversely proportional to the level of magnesium in the drinking water."
Source: http://www.mgwater.com/diabetes.shtml

In cases of type II diabetes where renal function is impaired, oral supplementation may be contraindicated, so transdermal magnesium supplementation could be recommended. Always consult with your GP before using any form of supplementation.

How can you help yourself?

Transdermal supplementation can be used in the form of a bath, foot bath, body spray, magnesium massage or Far Infrared Magnesium wrap. Magnesium baths and foot baths may be an excellent way to promote healing for diabetic ulcers and increasing sensitivity in the feet. As for frequency, daily applications of magnesium oil or magnesium baths/ foot baths may be very beneficial.

14. Obesity, weight problems

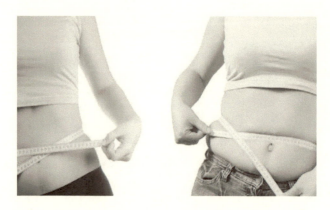

As can be seen from the analysis above, obesity and weight problems are directly linked to magnesium deficiency. Of course, it would be irresponsible of me to say that this is the only reason for obesity. If it were this simple, the problem of obesity would have been solved ages ago and we would all be healthy. Nevertheless, magnesium plays a major role in metabolising nutrients – fat, carbohydrates and proteins, so when there is not enough of it circulating in the body, nutrients don't get processed, so energy does not get produced in sufficient amounts for the body to function, leading to slowing down of metabolism. Moreover, magnesium deficiency leads to insulin resistance, which directly impacts on the metabolic processes and energy production, as is seen above.

How can you help yourself?

To correct the imbalance, daily magnesium supplementation is important, alongside healthy nutrition and exercise. Transdermal therapy is the fastest way to top up its content. Apply magnesium oil by hand, spray over the body or take baths and foot baths with magnesium salts – chloride, sulphate or Dead Sea salt. A Far Infrared Weight Loss wrap performed regularly could help to speed up the process. Not only will it deliver magnesium to the body in the quickest possible way, but will also promote sweating, which in turn helps to eliminate toxic waste.

15. Asthma

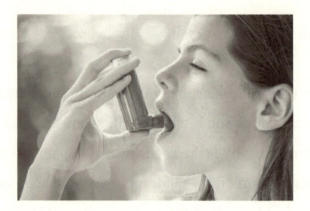

Asthma has been linked to magnesium deficiency in a wide variety of studies. Results of two such studies are described below. In the first study, Dead Sea water is used to relieve asthma symptoms. The Dead Sea is very rich in magnesium, which scientists believe explains the results.

Study 1:

Harari M, Barzillai R, Shani J.
The recognition of asthma as an inflammatory disease has led over the past 20 years to a major shift in its

pharmacotherapy. The previous emphasis on using relatively short-acting agents for relieving bronchospasms and for removing bronchial mucus has shifted toward long-term strategies with the use of inhaled corticosteroids, which successfully prevent and abolish airway inflammation. Because some of the biological, chemical, and immunological processes that characterize asthma also underlie arthritis and other inflammatory diseases, and because many of these conditions have been successfully treated for the past 40 years at the Dead Sea, we were not surprised to realize and record the significant improvement of an asthmatic condition after a 4-week stay at the Dead Sea: lung function was improved, the number and severity of attacks was reduced, and the efficacy of beta2-agonist treatments was improved. After reviewing the acute and chronic treatments of asthma in the clinic (including emergency rooms) with magnesium compounds, and the use of such salts as supplementary agents in respiratory diseases, we suggest that the improvement in the asthmatic condition at the Dead Sea may be due to absorption of this element through the skin and via the lungs, and due to its involvement in anti-inflammatory and vasodilatatory processes".

https://www.ncbi.nlm.nih.gov/pubmed/9777879?dopt=Abstract

Study 2:

Dr John Briffa says:

"Magnesium therapy was tried in a study published recently in the Journal of Asthma [1]. In it, 55 adults with mild-moderate asthma were treated with magnesium (170 mg, twice a day) or placebo over a period of 6.5 months. Individuals had their lung function tested using peak expiratory flow (the maximum speed air can be expelled from the lungs) as well as something known as the methacholine challenge test. Metacholine causes constriction of airways. In this test, subjects breathe in metacholine. The higher the dose of metacholine required, the less 'reactive' the airways would be judged to be.

Compared to those taking placebo, those taking magnesium saw significant improvement in both their peak expiratory flow rate and metacholine challenge results".
http://www.drbriffa.com/blog/2010/01/29/magnesium-therapy-found-to-benefit-asthmatics

What could be a possible explanation for the improvement? Marcela Davalos Bichara and Ran D. Goldman M.D. cite the following reasons:

"In vitro studies demonstrated the role of magnesium in the relaxation of bronchial cells. In smooth muscle, magnesium decreases intracellular calcium by blocking its entry and its release from the endoplasmic reticulum and by activating sodium-calcium pumps. Furthermore, inhibition of calcium's interaction with myosin results in muscle cell relaxation. Magnesium also stabilizes T cells and inhibits mast cell degranulation, leading to a reduction in inflammatory mediators. In cholinergic motor nerve terminals, magnesium depresses muscle fibre excitability by inhibiting acetylcholine release. Lastly, magnesium stimulates nitric oxide and prostacyclin synthesis, which might reduce asthma severity."

https://www.ncbi.nlm.nih.gov/pmc/articles/PMC2743582/

How can you help yourself?

Apart from intravenous injections of magnesium sulphate, regular magnesium supplementation could contribute not only to a lessening of symptoms, but also to a reduction of frequency of the attacks.

Taking daily magnesium sulphate or magnesium chloride baths, spraying magnesium oil on the body and having Far Infrared magnesium wraps once or twice a week could help to reduce inflammation of the airways and severity of asthma attacks.

16. Magnesium for girls and women

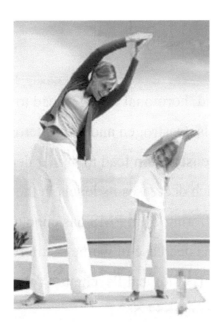

At every age of life, a woman's body requires lots of magnesium to function and stay healthy. Childhood, adolescence, pregnancy, menopause and maturity – all of these stages create their challenges and requirements.

Throughout the reproductive age, the body undergoes constant hormonal changes. Ovulation, menstruation, pregnancy, childbirth, lactation and menopause put a lot of strain on a woman's body. Hormone production puts a heavy requirement on magnesium. Magnesium deficiencies lead to hormonal imbalances, which in turn result in disturbances of important body processes.

On the other hand, hormonal changes lead to changes in magnesium levels. Oestrogen and progesterone rise during ovulation and menstruation lead to higher demands on magnesium, which decreases its levels in the body. A study of 19 women suffering from PMS has concluded that magnesium levels decrease in women-sufferers as opposed to non-sufferers. (Biological Psychiatry Volume 35, Issue 8, 15 April 1994, Pages 557-561).

We have all heard of women craving chocolate just before the period is due. Dark chocolate is abundant in magnesium, and the body instinctively chooses the food containing it. It has been said to help with cramps and mood swings associated with PMS. Magnesium is a natural relaxant, so is great for relieving menstrual cramps which are said to be linked to magnesium deficiency.

Pregnancy puts an enormous strain on the woman's body, with extra requirements of minerals not only for the mother but the foetus too. Magnesium deficiency in pregnancy may lead to a very dangerous condition called pre-eclampsia which may lead to eclampsia - both conditions are associated with dangerously high blood pressure. Magnesium Sulphate has been used in the treatment of women with pre-eclampsia for many decades. In hospitals, it is administered intravenously. However, many pregnant women use it transdermally, by taking Epsom Salt baths regularly.

Magnesium entering the mother's body invariably benefits the child. It has been suggested that prenatal magnesium administration may reduce the risk of cerebral palsy for very low birthweight babies. (Nelson K. Magnesium sulfate and risk of cerebral palsy in very-low-birth-weight infants. JAMA. 1996;276:1843–1844).

However, where magnesium is administered to a pregnant woman intravenously, it can also cause hypermagnesemia [too much magnesium – GSG] in babies with such symptoms as flaccidity, hyporeflexia, and respiratory depression. (Lipsitz PJ. The clinical and biochemical effects of excess magnesium in the newborn. Paediatrics. 1971;47:501–509). This has not been mentioned about transdermal magnesium applications where magnesium enters the body naturally.

A scientific study has shown that dietary magnesium deficiency in rats has resulted in a failure to lactate and impaired growth and development in their offspring. http://jn.nutrition.org/content/113/12/2421.full.pdf

This shows that magnesium is a crucial element which is required at various stages of a woman's life, especially during the reproductive phase.

How can you help yourself?

The best way to use Epsom salt is by having a bath with it.

Use 500g per bath, 2-3 times a week, for a profound therapeutic effect. Hand applications or spraying magnesium oil on the body daily is another option, and oral supplementation should be considered too.

17. Fertility & sexual health

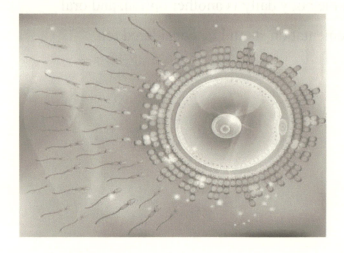

Magnesium is crucial for the production of healthy sperm and eggs, as well as for all the reproductive processes – ovulation, conception, gestation, birth, lactation, establishing of a bond between mother and baby, healthy sexual relationships.

"Sex, in particular, has become a major source of anxiety and stress for many of us and this is not all our fault... Magnesium is necessary for normal sexual functioning, yet is glossed over in its importance in nervous and endocrine function necessary for good sexual performance". (Mark Sircus, Transdermal Magnesium Therapy, 2007, p.234). Magnesium levels are very high in the semen – higher than in the blood serum. Infertile men have been found to have half the level of magnesium in their semen as fertile men (Mark Sircus, Transdermal Magnesium Therapy, 2007, p.235).

Magnesium affects the production and transmission of all hormones in the body – serotonin, thyroid, estrogen, testosterone, insulin, neurotransmitters, etc.

In his book, Dr Sircus plays special attention to the role of magnesium in the production of DHEA – dehydroepiandrosterone which "appears to protect every part of the body against the ravages of ageing" and is "flaunted as a "fountain of youth" (Mark Sircus, Transdermal Magnesium Therapy, 2007p.237, 241).

DHEA is a steroid hormone produced by the adrenal glands both in men and women. Its level peaks in puberty and drops in the early 30s. It is converted in the body into many hormones, including estrogen and testosterone. It affects muscle growth, libido, sperm production and much more.

The publicity of the age-defying effect of DHEA on the body has led to a surge in the population taking it as a synthetic supplement, says Dr Sircus, purchased both on prescription and over the counter. He points out many adverse effects resulting from such supplementation, including unwanted hair in women, acne, increased risk of ovarian cancer, breast cancer, prostate cancer in men, heart attacks).

At the same time, Dr Sircus points out that deficiency in DHEA leads not simply to ageing on all levels, but also "chronic inflammation, immune dysfunction, depression, rheumatoid arthritis, type 2 diabetes, greater risk of certain cancers, excess body fat, cognitive decline, heart disease in men, osteoporosis".

Erectile dysfunctions in men are closely related to magnesium deficiency. Dr Sircus points out that transdermal supplementation of magnesium leads to a boost of magnesium in the body and increase in DHEA and testosterone, which helps to improve the sexual function and libido, both in men and women.

Transdermal magnesium supplementation normalises levels of DHEA and boosts levels of testosterone in men and to a smaller extent in women. It balances the levels of estrogen and progesterone in women, thus reducing menopausal symptoms, menstrual problems, PMT, development of pre-eclampsia in pregnant women.

A boost in magnesium levels through transdermal supplementation is fast and free of side-effects which sometimes arise with oral supplementation. Because of the speed with which magnesium is replenished through transdermal procedures, the effects of it can be felt quickly on all levels, including reproductive the function both in men and women.

Dr Sircus writes, referring to a study in Japan: "In men, decreased levels of magnesium gives rise to vasoconstriction from increased thromboxane level, increased endothelial intracellular calcium, and decreased nitric oxide. This may lead to premature emission and ejaculation processes. Magnesium is also probably involved in semen transport." (Magnesium for Life, 2007, p.244)

A big revelation for me in Dr Sircus' book was information regarding the topical application of magnesium oil to reproductive organs regularly, especially just before having sex. Such applications would relax the tissues and quickly increase blood circulation in the area, both in men and women. It would also promote vaginal lubrication and relaxation of the muscles in the vagina, which would help eliminate the sensation of pain and discomfort during sex. In men, it would lead to a relaxation of the blood vessels supplying the penis, an increase in the blood flow and sensation in the area, and a stronger, longer-lasting erection.

Considering that the effect of such an application is so profound both in men and in women, it is difficult to understand why this has not been publicised on a much wider scale. The market is flooded with legally and illegally-produced medicines loaded with dangerous side-effects, and magnesium is not only safe to use in most cases, but is needed by the body in large quantities.

Transdermal applications increase absorption of magnesium into the body, dilate blood vessels, relax muscles and body tissues, increase peripheral circulation and improve tissue sensitivity and fluid secretions.

While there is much more to a satisfying sex life than an abundance of magnesium in the body, we need to remember that without the essential building blocks our bodies cannot function. Magnesium is one such very important component which we need in large quantities to help us live a long and happy life.

How can you help yourself?

Supplementation methods: oral, transdermal – bath, foot bath, topical (the genitals – dilute if required) and all-over applications of magnesium oil. Magnesium Massage and Far Infrared Magnesium wrap treatments can be used too.

18. Stretch marks, old scars

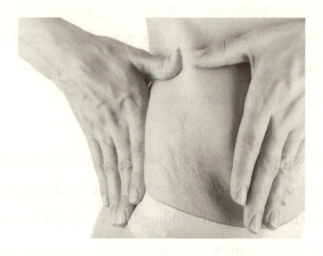

Stretch marks (striae distensae) happen as a result of rapid growth or weight gain. They look red, purple or white – depending on how old they are. The older the stretch marks, the lighter in colour. Pregnant women and teenage girls, as well as women who have had breast implants (especially of a large size), are especially vulnerable. While there is no guaranteed way to prevent or get rid of stretch marks, there are ways to minimise them.

First of all, it is important to remember that prevention is better than cure, so if a rapid body growth is expected, then one needs to prepare for it by improving the skin elasticity. This should be done by eating vitamin and mineral-rich food. The most important vitamins are A, B, C, D & E. The most important minerals to keep the skin supple are magnesium, selenium, sulphur, silica and zinc.

All of these vitamins and minerals are best taken in a food form. However, because it is required for so many body processes and is deficient in so many of us, I suggest supplementing magnesium additionally by using magnesium salts transdermally, which means applying magnesium oil on the skin.

Regular applications of magnesium oil on the skin will increase its elasticity, which in turn will help to prevent stretch marks from developing. Magnesium will also relax the skin layers and promote healing of existing stretch marks. The same applies to old scar tissue. While it is not going to make stretch marks and scars disappear, regularly massaging the area with magnesium oil could help reduce their prominence and appearance, as well as prevent deterioration of the tissue.

How can you help yourself?

I suggest applying magnesium oil on the skin daily for best results. The reason for it is that a bath has a much lower concentration of magnesium in it than magnesium oil applied directly on the skin.

A Far Infrared Magnesium Wrap used once or twice a week will help to boost magnesium in the body even more, which will promote skin elasticity and help reduce stretch marks. Of course, like anything in this book, this is not guaranteed but is well worth trying.

19. Heavy metal & radioactive toxicity

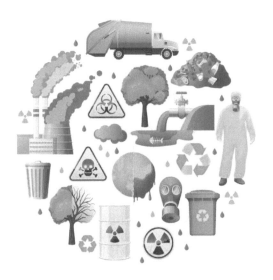

Since the subject of the nuclear fallout from the earthquake in Japan is going to be at the top of the list for all health-conscious people and health professionals for an indefinite time, I think it is important to spread the message of the importance of minerals in protecting us all from radiation, as well as general heavy metal toxicity of the environment we now live in. It is no secret that the economic progress has led to alarming rises in the number, as well as levels, of heavy metals in everything around us, including food, water and air.

In a normal, healthy environment with nutritionally abundant uncontaminated soil and clean air and water, the body would receive all the nutrients it needs and perform all the cleaning and detoxification procedures efficiently, without the need for any interference from our part.

However, we do not live in an ideal environment, and unfortunately, things are not getting any better, which means that our body needs help – in the form of mineral supplementation –to help it to detoxify from heavy metals.

Minerals play a vital role not only in detoxification from heavy metals, but they also help to protect us from further radioactive damage. Popular thinking is that radiation protection mostly involves using iodine, so iodine supplements have been taken in large numbers recently, by those who need it and those who don't, while supplementation in such vital minerals as magnesium and selenium is being often overlooked.

Magnesium supports all the body systems and detoxification processes. It provides the body with the energy it needs to ensure the elimination of toxins. Magnesium is an integral part of glutathione - a detoxifying agent which protects the body from oxidative damage. It binds toxins into soluble substances excreting them with urine through the kidneys. When magnesium is deficient, the body cannot produce sufficient glutathione, leading to cellular damage from free radicals, which leaves them exposed to further radioactive damage. Liver, kidneys, the heart, the lungs, as well as other organs of the body all have glutathione, and with magnesium deficiency, all of these vital organs are exposed to radiation. Magnesium plays a vital role in detoxification of the body from mercury, cadmium, lead and aluminium.

How can you help yourself?

The best way to supplement magnesium in the home environment is through the skin. Magnesium chloride is the most easily absorbed form of magnesium. So I can suggest using magnesium massage, magnesium spray, magnesium bath, foot bath, magnesium wrap, and any form of magnesium application you can think of.

Consider including zinc, selenium and iodine in your diet, as well as sulphur-rich foods such as garlic, onion, cabbage, Brussel sprouts, apricots, green vegetables, herbs and algae such as seaweed, Sun Chlorella, spirulina and coriander. Other transdermal detoxification procedures such as clay and zeolite baths or a course of Far Infrared Clay Detox wraps will help to kick-start the detox process.

20. Sport

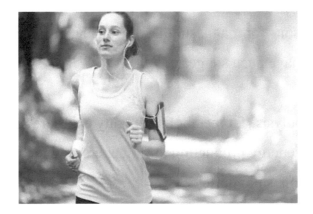

Athletes are especially prone to magnesium losses and resulting deficiency, which can lead to reduced performance, muscle rigidity, tetany, cramps, decreased endurance, general weakness, as well as an array of cardiovascular problems such as an increase in blood pressure, arrhythmia and rigidity of the blood vessels.

While short high-intensity exercise leads to an increase of magnesium levels (hypermagnesemia), due to a shift of magnesium from cells into plasma as a result of acidosis and a general decrease of plasma levels, prolonged exercise leads to a depletion of plasma magnesium as well, which can result in hypomagnesemia.

A few reasons for magnesium losses during prolonged sports activities have been suggested:

1. Lipolysis (fat metabolism). Fatty acids are mobilised for energy production during exercise which leads to magnesium deficiency.

2. General physical and psychological stress on all body systems during prolonged exercise.

3. Loss of magnesium through sweating – this normally happens in humid hot conditions.

4. A loss of magnesium in urine during intensive short-term exercise activities.

Magnesium losses are especially substantial during periods of training for sporting events. "Several studies indicate that there is a sustained fall in plasma Mg concentration after strenuous exercise and that hypomagnesaemia either persists or worsens during a season of training 21,46,47,48, a sound reason for looking more carefully at the Mg intake of athletes. A recent longitudinal study of a group of medium-distance runners carried out over a training season also demonstrated plasma Mg reductions during the competition period, although there were no variations in erythrocyte Mg. Since both their energy intake and their workload remained more or less constant during the study, a relationship can be established between plasma Mg changes and the stress of the competition period 4" (Y. Rayssiguier1, C. Y. Guezennec2, and J. Durlach3, New experimental and clinical data on the relationship between magnesium and sport, http://www.mgwater.com/dur18.shtml

Magnesium deficiency may play a role in the sudden death syndrome in sportspeople resulting from a cardiac arrest (heart attack). As has been mentioned earlier, a fall in magnesium levels in sportspeople can lead to an increase in cholesterol, blood sugar levels, and rigidity of blood vessels which in turn results in an increase in blood pressure and may in some cases explain sudden death in athletes.

All this brings us to a conclusion that it is extremely

important to replenish magnesium levels in athletes, especially during prolonged sporting activities and competitions, to prevent a slump in energy levels, general fatigue, reduction in performance, muscle tension, aches and pains and speed up the recovery.

It is also important to remember that magnesium plays a major role in the healing and restoration of elasticity of the body tissues after a sports injury. Of course, with all fresh injuries, it is important to follow the protocol and apply cold compresses at the beginning to minimise the damage. Once it starts to heal, magnesium applications will speed things up and repair the damage to the area, as well as help to restore its function.

How can you help yourself?

Magnesium oil applications all over the body, especially after a strenuous exercise and events such as marathon runs and cycling competitions would do wonders for sportspeople.

A magnesium bath would relax the muscles bringing required magnesium to the system. Magnesium footbaths would benefit runners especially.

Take oral supplements if you exercise a lot since your requirement in magnesium would be much higher than for a non-sporty person.

21. Allergies & chemical sensitivities

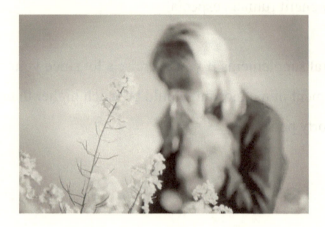

Many researchers believe that food allergies and chemical sensitivities are connected with the body producing too little stomach acid, which leaves some of the food undigested. Stomach acid does not only break down food in the stomach. It also creates an environment for the beneficial gut flora to function. When there is not enough of it, the "friendly" bacteria greatly diminish in numbers, which leads to malabsorption of nutrients in the intestinal tract.

The symptoms of low stomach acid are gas, belching, bloating, diarrhoea and IBS. In the stomach, it leads to acid reflux or heartburn. Yes, it may be surprising, but low acid is responsible for heartburn, even though we are conditioned to believe that it is the high content of hydrochloric acid that causes it. So taking antacids in such cases would make things worse, not better!

Indigested food triggers a response from the body defences which start producing histamine in large amounts in response to what the body "believes" to be foreign matter (undigested food). When it happens regularly, food sensitivities and even allergies develop.

Of course, the subject of allergic reactions is a complex one and is under constant research. However, it is important to investigate if you suffer from low stomach acidity before you embark on any treatment. A nutrition adviser or dietician should be able to help adjust your diet to correct this imbalance.

Allergies and food sensitivities often show on the skin as eczema and dermatitis, as well as spots and rashes of various appearances.

How can you help yourself?

Magnesium has a proven antihistamine action calming down a body response to potential allergens. If you have low stomach acid already, taking magnesium supplements may make the problem worse. In this case, transdermal magnesium applications will be the best option. Apply it by hand, as a spray, take magnesium salt baths with magnesium chloride, Epsom salt or Dead Sea salt, or try a Far Infrared Magnesium wrap for quick delivery of magnesium to the body tissues and organs.

If you suffer from Hay Fever, you may also benefit from nasal rinses. Dilute about 1 teaspoon (5g) of Himalayan salt in 100ml of water. Use a pipette or a nasal irrigation kit to rinse your nose 3-4 times a day on the days when there is high pollen count. We are not using magnesium salts for this purpose because magnesium is a natural relaxant, so will expand the vessels in the nasal passages even further, thus making the symptoms worse.

22. Ageing skin & wrinkles

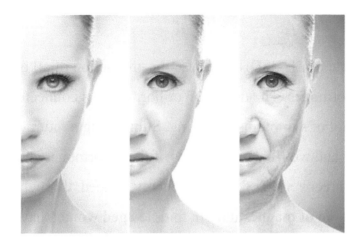

In his book "Holy Water, Sacred Oil", Dr Norman Shealy draws a strong correlation between magnesium levels and DHEA levels. He also states that when body cells have sufficient magnesium in them, it begins to naturally produce DHEA.

DHEA

Since DHEA comprises the basic bio-marker for ageing, the long-term use of large doses of magnesium in an available form will significantly bring up DHEA levels and thus produce true Age Reversal results. Dr Shealy refers to DHEA as the Master Hormone.

Adequate levels of DHEA cause the production of all of the other hormones. The depletion of hormones is connected with a lot of symptoms of ageing. Stimulating a return to healthy and well-balanced levels of these hormones can give rise to a recovering of youthful energy. Indeed, through the application of magnesium oil, middle-aged women have described complete reprieve from menopausal symptoms and some have even returned to their menstrual cycle.

Dr Shealy has stated that once anyone starts regular use of Magnesium Oil, the ageing process is arrested and true age reversal begins. There is also a trend to supplement DHEA directly, but it is deemed too controversial and benefits unproven, with some researchers citing no direct improvement as a result of supplementation while noting serious side-effects.

Even if you don't believe in DHEA and its effects,

magnesium is needed for the maintenance of skin elasticity and production of collagen. If there is a magnesium-calcium imbalance in favour of calcium, as is the case in most people of advanced age, the dermal layer loses its elasticity because fibres become calcified. If magnesium is not being supplemented, this process continues resulting in the face and other muscles contracting while fibres supporting the skin lose their elasticity. All of this makes the skin aged and wrinkled.

Direct magnesium application on the skin regularly can start reversing the damage done to the skin, resulting in an overall improvement of its condition and elasticity. And of course, the body benefits from such applications in many other ways.

How can you help yourself?

Apply magnesium oil on the skin daily. Rub magnesium oil on the face and scalp, as well as arms, shoulders, neck and chest. Make magnesium-based warm compresses and masks. If you want to notice the results, take pictures of yourself when you start the procedures and then 3 months later. See if you notice any difference!

Eating lots of antioxidant-rich foods, cutting down on sugar, alcohol, cigarettes, junk food and too much sun, drinking plenty of water, making sure that you sleep enough hours every day and exercising will help even further.

23. Acne

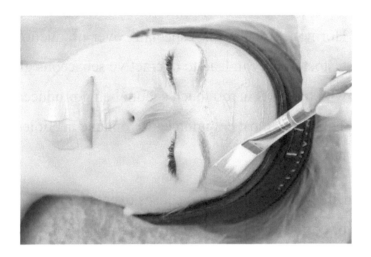

Acne Vulgaris is a condition caused by blockages of hair follicles due to too much sebum production. The area becomes inflamed because of bacteria proliferation in the blocked follicle, which results in acne.

Acne affects people of all sexes and ages – male and female, babies, teenagers, adults and even the elderly. Babies can get hormones passed from their mothers which can result in an outbreak of acne. Older people can get acne alongside wrinkles too. However, it is a teenage acne that is most common.

Common causes of acne include:

1. Hormone imbalances, especially over-production of testosterone, can lead to overactive sebaceous glands which results in too much sebum being produced. This is the most common cause of acne in adolescent boys and girls.

2. Stress. Prolonged stress causes excessive production of cortisol which interferes with the control of blood sugar and leads to hyperactivity of sebaceous glands and acne.

3. Poor nutrition, especially excessive consumption of sugary food and drinks. This too creates imbalances in the blood sugar levels and production of too much sebum.

4. Some people react badly to milk. It is believed that this can be caused by hormones in milk.

5. Toxicity resulting from an intake of toxins in food, water, medicines, heavy metals, alcohol, drugs and

tobacco – upsets hormonal activity in the body and can lead to acne.

Medical treatment for acne includes antibiotics, drugs such as Roaccutane, retinoid containing creams, over-the-counter gels and ointments. While antibiotics show good results, they disrupt digestion and body's defences which can lead more acne once the treatment is over, as well as other side-effects including hair loss, dry skin, headaches and depression.

How can you help yourself?

Magnesium supplementation is important at all stages of life. It helps to relax the nervous system which in turn helps to balance hormones, sugar and regulate the production of sebum.

Oral supplementation can be combined with transdermal. For transdermal supplementation use magnesium oil spray, rub or a massage, magnesium-based face masks, magnesium baths and foot baths. Also, you could make a face wash using 1 part of magnesium oil to 4 parts of water. Wash the face with the solution twice a day, apply coconut oil to soothe the skin and help to protect it.

Just to dispel the myth – oil is not bad for the skin. The skin produces its oil called sebum to protect itself from infection. It is when there is too much of it getting produced that it blocks the pores causing acne. So don't be afraid of applying coconut or jojoba oil after a mask/ treatment.

Other things to consider:

1. Eat well. A diet low in refined carbohydrates and sugar, high in what is good for the body – fibre, vegetables, good fats and protein will help to keep hormones in balance. Ensure you eat a lot of antioxidant-rich food.

2. Exercise, especially outside. In my opinion, a brisk walk in the fresh air offers a lot more benefits than sweating in a smelly gym.

3. Recognise what makes you stressed and develop your stress management strategy. Meditate. Take on a hobby. Read. Meet people. Do what makes you feel good.

4. Sleep your hours. It is impossible to overestimate the benefits of a good night's sleep. Go to bed before midnight, to make sure that you benefit from the sleep hormone melatonin which balances the immune system and hormones.

5. Drink lots of water to flush toxins out of the body. Toxic waste interferes with how we feel and our skin health.

6. Green clay masks work well for acne since they work by cleansing the pores of impurities, killing bacteria. Apply once or twice per week adding magnesium oil for more effect. Tone and condition the skin with lemon water and coconut or jojoba oil afterwards.

24. Mental health

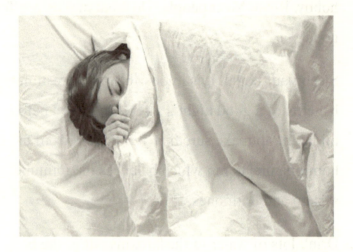

Magnesium is a mineral which promotes relaxation not only of muscles but also of nerve tissue and the brain, which is very important when addressing mental health issues. Scientific research has established that people suffering from mental problems have one thing in common – magnesium deficiency.

While magnesium is not the only answer to treating mental health problems, it is nevertheless a major piece in the puzzle. Magnesium plays a crucial role in the release and uptake of serotonin by the brain cells. When there is sufficient magnesium in the body we produce enough serotonin and are in balance. Magnesium deficiency, on the other hand, causes not only serotonin deficit, but also anxiety, worry, insomnia, nervous tension and general psychological stress which in turn make mental health problems worse.

Like with other issues, mental health issues have various causes. Nevertheless, magnesium intake and applications provide a mineral which is responsible for over 300 reactions in the body including the production of neurotransmitters, enzymes and hormones responsible for maintaining sound mental health.

Magnesium supplementation has demonstrated excellent results in children with ADHD and Autism. It has a lot of benefits for people with a variety of mental health problems acting as a calming and stabilising mineral.

A study in the US established a link between hypomagnesemia and eating disorders, as well as general

mental state. 25% of people suffering from bulimia who took part in the research had low magnesium levels. Magnesium supplementation showed considerable improvement of symptoms associated with the condition.
http://www.drrichardhall.com/Articles/hypomagnesemia.pdf

How can you help yourself?

Taking magnesium supplements orally will certainly help to raise magnesium levels. Transdermal delivery of this mineral works faster though, so using magnesium baths, applying magnesium oil by hand or a spray and even having Far Infrared Magnesium wraps regularly will help to restore magnesium in the body to an optimal level and contribute to the restoration of good mental health.

25. Cancer

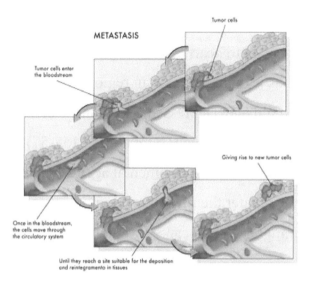

I cannot stress highly enough how important magnesium is not only in the prevention but also the treatment of cancer. It has been researched that countries with a low magnesium level in the soil have a higher incidence of cancer among the population. Another factor is nutrition and exercise - countries with a high level of obesity, caused by high consumption of alcohol and sugar/fat-rich foods, combined with a low level of activity, count a high number of people suffering from cancer, which is also linked to magnesium deficiency as one of the symptoms. Below I am reposting an article which I wrote some time ago.

"Cancer is second to heart disease as a cause of death in the aged, and thus is more common in regions where more people reach old age. Depressed B-cell and T-cell immunologic function, occur with ageing. (55-57) Also, the longer the exposure to environmental agents with oncogenic potential, the greater the risk of developing cancer".
http://www.mgwater.com/cancer.shtml

Worldwide studies have established that the cancer rate increases with the decreased magnesium content of water and soil.

On May 19, 1931, Dr Schrumpf-Pierron presented a paper entitled "On the Cause of the Rarity of Cancer in Egypt". In it he concluded:

1. "Cancer for Egypt is about one-tenth that of Europe and America.

2. In Egypt, cancer is less frequent in-country fellahin than in the Egyptians who live in the towns and who have adopted Europeanized dietary habits.
3. The degree of malignancy of Egyptian cancers is less than that of European cancers. They develop less quickly and have less of a tendency to invade neighbouring tissues.
4. The type of cancer which is the most frequent in all the countries rich in cancer is the cancer of the digestive, tract, which represents 40 to 50 per cent of all cancers. In the case of Egyptians, this type of cancer is remarkably rare; in the country fellahin, practically nonexistent".

http://www.mgwater.com/rod02.shtml

He concluded that the prevalence of potassium in the soils of European countries and their diets and not enough magnesium leads to an increased risk of cancer. In Egypt, both the soil and diet is rich in magnesium, and for this reason, he saw it as the main factor in the very low cancer rate among Egyptians.

"An intoxication of potash - an excess of potash poisons - can "kill" the soil where the food is grown. It poisons the plants, then man. Besides, several other authorities have already accused potash of producing cancer. Theis and Benedikt, as well as Mentrier, have already stated that the higher amount of potash in cancerous tissue, which is a radioactive body, would cause the multiplication of cancerous cells".
http://www.mgwater.com/rod02.shtml

In her article "Magnesium in Oncogenesis and in Anti-Cancer Treatment: Interaction with Minerals and Vitamins", Mildred S. Seelig, M.D., M.P.H. says that magnesium deficiency can both decrease and paradoxically protect against cancer. For example, magnesium supplementation of those who are magnesium-deficient (e.g. chronic alcoholics) may protect them against developing some tumours.

"Optimal Mg intake may be prophylactic against initiation of some neoplasms. Since cancer cells have high metabolic requirements, it is not indicated (alone) in the treatment of cancer."

The author then points out a correlation between water hardness and longevity: "Since environmental factors have been judged likely to contribute to most human cancers, it is worth effort to ascertain if there are protective geochemical agents. Determining what it is in different geographic regions that affects life expectancy, provides one approach. The largest area in the United States of America (USA) with increased longevity is in the north and central plains; the largest area with decreased longevity is in the south-eastern coastal area. These are hard and soft water regions, respectively".

Worldwide studies have established a reverse correlation of magnesium deficiency in soil and prevalence of certain types of cancer.

"A Russian report showed that stomach cancer is four times more common (40/100,000) in the Ukraine where the Mg content of soil and drinking water is low than it is in Armenia (10/100,000) where the Mg content is more than twice as high. (14,66-68) A more recent morphologic and statistical analysis of neoplastic deaths in two Polish communities(69) disclosed a nearly three-fold higher death rate in the one in a low soil Mg area (27%) than in the one with high soil Mg (10%). The malignancies accounting for the differences were mainly adeno- and squamous cell carcinomas in the gastrointestinal tract (61.3%) and respiratory system (22.3%)".

"Correlation of high rates of leukemia with low levels of Mg in soil and water is concordant with experiments showing that chronic Mg deficiency can cause lymphosarcomas and leukemia in rats".

"Connective tissue, made up of fibroblastic cells that produced collagen type III, proliferated in the intestines of rats maintained on severely Mg deficient diets for at least 8 weeks. A less Mg-restricted diet did not evoke such tumors.

She goes on to conclude: "Despite provocative findings that suggest that Mg deficiency might be implicated in aspects of pathogenesis and treatment of neoplasms, there are many unknowns. Investigation of these questions might lead to means to prevent lympholeukemias, or possibly of immuno-incompetence. Whether higher Mg intakes might be protective against oncogens in humans as it is in some animal models deserves study".

http://www.mgwater.com/cancer.shtml

Due to a magnesium deficiency in most soils, we do not receive even a fraction of this vital mineral of what is required by the body to keep us healthy. This makes it very important to supplement magnesium in other ways. The best way to supplement magnesium in home conditions is by using magnesium oil – applying it on the skin daily, either by spraying it or rubbing it in with a hand.

How can you help yourself?

If you decide to go for oral supplementation, then use an absorbable form of it – like magnesium citrate or magnesium orotate. Both of these ensure that magnesium does not irritate the gut and that it gets absorbed into the system instead of being eliminated from the body.

The fastest and safest supplementation method for cancer sufferers is transdermal. Apply magnesium oil all over the body regularly, by hand or as a spray. Take regular baths and foot baths with magnesium chloride or sulphate. Book magnesium massage or Far Infrared Magnesium wrap (ask your doctor if it is ok to do so).

How to Make Magnesium Oil at Home

Magnesium chloride salt exists in nature as magnesium brine. It is found in deep underground deposits – down to 2km deep in some cases, and in seawater. Much of the seawater magnesium chloride is obtained from the Dead Sea.

Most of the underground magnesium chloride comes from the Eurasian deposits, stretching from Siberia to Europe. The brine is often called "magnesium oil", and the salt is commonly known as "flakes".

Magnesium chloride flakes are 47% magnesium chloride and about 50.5% water. A 33% solution means that there will be 33% magnesium chloride.

Although it is best to use magnesium oil which is made from a brine, sometimes it is not an option. In such cases, you can make your magnesium oil. Here is a rough guide on how to make it.

100 grams of flakes (which contain 50.5 grams of water) will need an extra 42 grams of water. (1g of water equals 1ml of water). The 47 grams of magnesium chloride will then be dissolved in 142 grams of solution, giving the 33% strength that is required. This can be scaled up to a convenient batch size – every kilogram of flakes will require 420 grams of water to be added. This will produce a concentrated magnesium oil solution. It will take a while to

dissolve, but you can warm it up to speed up the process.

I use a simpler method of preparing my magnesium oil. I add 1 part of warm water to 1 part of magnesium flakes by weight. This produces a less concentrated solution, but it dissolves a lot more quickly. It is also better for dry and sensitive skin types.

Magnesium-rich foods

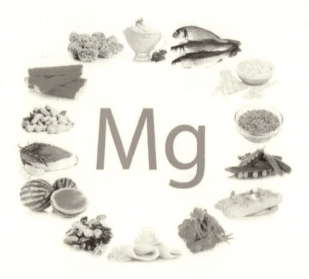

Having talked at length about magnesium supplementation, it is important to mention that eating magnesium-rich food should be your priority to keep magnesium levels high at all times.

Most of the magnesium we have in our body comes from food and food supplements. Magnesium-rich food products include:

- Dark leafy greens (spinach, kale)
- Wild (not farmed) fish and seafood
- Nuts (Brazil nuts, almonds, peanuts, walnuts)
- Dried fruit (dates, figs, apricots)
- Black-eyed beans
- Pumpkin, sunflower and other seeds
- Yoghurt
- Whole grains
- Dark chocolate
- Bananas
- Avocados
- Broccoli
- Seafood
- Eggs
- Watermelons
- Yellow corn
- Dry roasted soybeans
- Coriander
- Artichokes.

Conclusion

In this book, I have listed only 25 most common conditions which benefit from magnesium supplementation. This list only touches briefly on a very big subject. There are many more problems which can and are helped by introducing magnesium to the body. It was not my purpose to list them all here. My goal was to bring the subject of magnesium supplementation to a wider public. If you want to learn more, I suggest again that you take a look at my blog – https://magnesiumoil.org.uk.

Further Information & Links

Get a FREE copy of the "Mineral Healing" report:

https://purenaturecures.com/

Read more about the treatments and courses offered by Pure Nature Cures:

https://courses.purenaturecures.com/

Check out my other books and courses from the Mineral Healing series:

https://amazon.com/author/galinastgeorge

Read more about magnesium for health:

https://magnesiumoil.org.uk

Email:

support@purenaturecures.com

Made in United States
Troutdale, OR
12/28/2023

16490876R00083